DO YOU WANT TO BE WELL AGAIN?

*Thoughts and prayers
at times of sickness*

Johnny Doherty, CSsR

First published 2005 *by*
Veritas Publications
7/8 Lower Abbey Street
Dublin 1
Ireland
Email publications@veritas.ie
Website www.veritas.ie

10 9 8 7 6 5 4 3 2 1

ISBN 1 85390 862 2

A catalogue record for this book is available from the British Library.

Psalms taken from *The Psalms: A New Translation* © The Grail (England) 1963.

Printed in the Republic of Ireland by Betaprint.

Veritas books are printed on paper made from the wood pulp of managed forests. For every tree felled, at least one tree is planted, thereby renewing natural resources.

To Annie and Mickey Doherty, my parents.
They taught me so much about life and love.

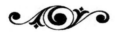

CONTENTS

FOREWORD BY FRANCIS HARTLEY

In April 2004 I was called for an operation to have my gall bladder removed. This is normally a fairly routine operation with just the usual difficulties of any minor surgery. However, for me it was different because I suffer from a serious lung disease and there was a strong possibility that my lungs could collapse during the operation and I would be in danger of dying. Thank God, as you can see it worked out alright and I am still very much alive!

For over a year the doctors and other medical personnel in two hospitals in Belfast prepared me for the gall bladder operation. That was a very difficult period for me. There were times when I thought I might not get as far as being operated on, times when I felt like I was going to die at any moment. I was very frightened. Other times I wasn't sure I wanted to live as I got so tired of being sick. I was frustrated and angry. And there were times when I felt good, times when I could have some hope that the future would be OK. In all of those times I wanted to pray because I knew how much I needed the company of God. Yet prayer became very difficult for me. I am the kind of person who likes to talk to God, but the words would not come. I tried a few books of prayer, but they were of little help to me.

Through all of this time I had wonderful support from my sisters and brothers, my nieces and nephews, and some friends. One of those friends is Fr Johnny Doherty to whom I spoke about the struggle I was having with prayer and the anguish I was in because of it. He began to write some of the reflections and prayers that are in this book to see how they would help. I immediately began to find them of immense value. I began to feel the presence of Jesus with me through the pain and suffering, in my moments of darkness, in the times when I was frightened. By the time I went for the operation he had just ten prayers written, but these helped me to face the operation without any fear because I knew that however it turned out I was going to be alright.

I am glad he has continued writing these reflections and now they are available to you in this publication. I encourage you to read them and choose the ones you find helpful at any particular time. I hope you will get as much comfort and strength from these as I did and that you will also be brought safely through your illness knowing the presence of Christ and the love that God has for you.

Jesus said to his disciples: 'Peace I bequeath to you, my own peace I give you, a peace the world cannot give, this is my gift to you. Do not let your hearts be troubled or afraid.' (John, 15, 27)

INTRODUCTION: COME TO ME

Jesus said: 'Come to me, all you who labour and are overburdened, and I will give you rest. Shoulder my yoke and learn from me, for I am gentle and humble of heart, and you will find rest for your souls! Yes, my yoke is easy and my burden light.' (Mt. 11, 28-30)

Reflection One of the wonderful features of the Gospels is the number of stories of healing we find there. Between the four Gospels and the Acts of the Apostles there are thirty-one different stories. Some of these are repeated in slightly different ways in two or three of the Gospels. This would indicate that healing is one of the major desires in the heart of Jesus and one of the main effects of his salvation for us.

However, Jesus did not come to change the patterns of human life. Those are the same now as they always were and will be until the end of time. One of those patterns is that we all grow older and that will not change no matter how much we might want it to! Another pattern is that there will always be people who are better than us in all kinds of ways; there will be others who are better off than we are, who have more talent than we have, who are more popular than we are, and so on. And one of the normal patterns of human life is sickness, suffering and disease. What Jesus offers us is not so much to be freed from all of these, but to be freed from the destructive effects that each of these can have on our human spirit. Illness and suffering especially can easily destroy us by taking away our peace of mind, by robbing us of hope, by making us so preoccupied with ourselves that we cannot think of others in love and care for them.

At all of these times when our spirit is in danger of despondency or despair we can listen to those wonderful words of Jesus: 'Come to me all you who labour and are overburdened and I will give you rest.' Just by letting those words sound in our hearts, we can feel that sense of rest take over in us. 'Shoulder my yoke and learn from me, for I am gentle and humble of heart, and you will find rest for your souls' – feel any tension that may be in you because of illness melt down into the gentle embrace of Christ as he hangs on the Cross to set us free. 'Yes, my yoke is easy and my burden is light' – on your own the weight of what you are suffering may feel too much for you to bear, but Jesus offers to carry that burden with you, and at times for you, so that your suffering can get caught up in his and become powerful for the salvation of the world.

Prayer Jesus, Son of God and Son of Mary, in your Passion and death on the Cross, you entered into the very depths of human suffering. Be with me now in the pain and suffering I am going through. Help me to listen to your invitation to let you journey with me through this time so that I may find the fulfilment of your promise in my life and that I might find rest for my soul. Gather my sufferings into yours and let me find gentleness and awe in the depths of my heart. Amen.

Soul of Christ, sanctify me,
Body of Christ save me.
Blood of Christ, inebriate me.
Water from the side of Christ wash me.
Passion of Christ, strengthen me.
O good Jesus, hear me.
Within your wounds hide me
Permit me not to be separated from you.
From the malignant enemy defend me.
In the hour of my death call me
And bid me come to you,
That with your saints I may praise you
For ever and ever. Amen.

NO ONE GOES AWAY DISAPPOINTED
A Number of Cures

At sunset all those who had friends suffering from diseases of one kind or another brought them to him (Jesus), and laying his hands on each he cured them. (Lk. 4, 40)

Reflection In the Gospels, many of those whom Jesus healed came to him themselves. Those who loved them, however, brought others to him. In both situations Jesus responded with love and with power. And that is true for us today. We can bring one another to him in our hearts and in our prayer, assured that he will listen to us and respond to us. We often feel helpless in the presence of the illness of someone we love dearly. We don't have to be like that as we have the most wonderful resource of healing for them that could ever be imagined. The scene we find in the above short Gospel reading is very reminiscent of a place like Lourdes where countless people with every sort of illness and disease gather, most of them brought there by their immediate family or by their faith family. There is a longing in the hearts of everyone present for Christ to lay his hands on each one and no one goes away disappointed.

Prayer God of compassion and love, we thank you for the extraordinary gift of Jesus, your Son, given to us as the sign of your love and as our constant companion, especially in times of sickness. Help me to know his presence now and to be comforted by that knowledge. When I feel frightened, help me to turn to him. When I feel alone, help me to be aware of him. And when I feel despair, help me to trust him so that even in my darkest times I can say with St Paul: 'I live, now not I, but Christ lives in me'. Amen.

Psalm 19
May the Lord answer in time of trial;
May the name of Jacob's God protect you.

May he send you help from his shrine
And give you support from Sion.
May he remember all your offerings
And receive your sacrifice with favour.

May he give you your heart's desire
And fulfil every one of your plans.
May we ring out our joy at your victory
And rejoice in the name of our God.
May the Lord grant all your prayers.

HEALING ADDICTIONS
Cure of a Blind Man at Bethsaida

They came to Bethsaida, and some people brought to Jesus a blind man whom they begged him to touch. He took the blind man by the hand and led him outside the village. Then putting spittle on his eyes and laying his hands on him, he asked, 'Can you see anything?' The man, who was beginning to see, replied, 'I can see people; they look like trees to me, but they are walking about'. Then he laid his hands on him again and he saw clearly; he was cured, and he could see everything clearly and distinctly. And Jesus sent him home, saying, 'Do not even go into the village'. (Mk. 8, 22-26)

Reflection A form of illness that we don't often think of as an illness is addiction. There are many of these, some much more harmful to health and well-being than others, but all of them coming from a certain blindness to the reality of what is happening. Well-known addictions are to alcohol, drugs, gambling, tobacco, sex. More recent addictions are to chat lines and website pornography.

Every addiction has a serious effect on the human person. Some of them, like smoking and alcoholism, affect a person's physical health; others, like alcoholism, gambling or sex addiction, can affect people's relationships. While more again affect people's minds, turning them into very self-centred people. All addictions need to be attended to in the name of personal health as well as social well-being.

Alcoholics Anonymous was the first group to tackle this personal and social illness and they showed clearly that addictions could be overcome. However, their first principle is that we cannot be healed by our own power. We need to acknowledge and call on 'A Higher Power'. As Christians we know this Higher Power as God made visible in Christ Jesus.

The acknowledgement of the Higher Power is only the first of twelve steps to recovery and will fail without the implementation of the other eleven. Most groups that have been founded for recovery from other addictions follow the same principles. And the great thing is that they work. It is like the man in the story above. He was only gradually healed. But each step took him closer to a full cure.

Prayer God our Creator, our Redeemer, our Sanctifier, without you nothing is possible. Help us all to know our need of you and your total desire to be with us to bring us to the fullness of life. We pray for all people who are caught up in addictions that are harmful to their health of body or mind or that are damaging or even destroying their family relationships. Help each one to come to her/his senses, to take responsibility for her/his actions, to acknowledge you as the one who can set her/him free through the gift of courage to take the addiction in hand. Bless all those who suffer from having an addict as part of their lives. Help them to seek out the support they need to enable them to handle their situation properly in love. And bless all the support groups for addicts, that the work they do may be greatly blessed and that very many people may be restored to health. We make our prayer through Christ, our Lord. Amen.

Psalm 118

I call with all my heart; Lord hear me,
I will keep your commands.
I call upon you, save me
and I will do your will.

I rise before dawn and cry for help,
I hope in your word.
My eyes watch through the night
to ponder your promise.

In your love hear my voice, O Lord:
give me life by your decrees.
Those who harm me unjustly draw near:
they are far from your law.

But you, O Lord, are close:
your commands are truth.
Long have I known that your will
is established forever.

THE GENTLENESS OF CHRIST

Cure of a Leper

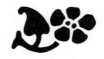

Now Jesus was in one of the towns when a man appeared, covered with leprosy. Seeing Jesus he fell on his face and implored him. 'Sir', he said, 'if you want to you can cure me.' Jesus stretched out his hand, touched him and said, 'Of course I want to. Be cured!' And the leprosy left him at once. He ordered him to tell no one. 'But go and show yourself to the priest and make the offering for your healing as Moses prescribed it, as evidence for them.'

His reputation continued to grow, and large crowds would gather to hear him and to have their sickness cured, but he would always go off to some place where he could be alone and pray. (Lk. 5, 12-16)

Reflection Leprosy was a terrible disease in the time of Jesus. It caused awful physical suffering for those who contracted it. But it also caused even worse social suffering as people with leprosy were regarded as outcasts and no one was allowed to approach those who had the disease in case it would spread and decimate the entire population.

Jesus broke through the taboos of his time and not only spoke to this man, but also touched him, thereby running the risk of becoming an outcast himself. We can hear the compassion and love in the conversation between Jesus and this man. At this moment he was the only important consideration in the heart of Jesus. The man cries out in anguish: 'If you want to, you can cure me'. And Jesus speaks with incredible gentleness: 'Of course I want to. Be cured'.

As you come to Jesus in your heart right now listen for that same compassion and love and gentleness in the heart of Jesus as he touches you and holds you in his warm embrace and speaks to your heart: 'Of course I want everything that is good for you. Trust me and together we will come through this difficult time for you and for those who love you.'

Prayer Father of love, I thank you for all the ways you show your love in my life. I thank you most of all for Jesus, your Son, who is given to us as the greatest sign of how much you love us. Be with me now at this time of my illness and fill my heart with peace and confidence. And bless all those who care for me and who are anxious during this time of my illness. May they find you more fully in their own lives. Amen.

Sacred Heart of Jesus, I place all my trust in you.

Psalm 53

O God, save me by your name,
by your power uphold my cause.
O God, hear my prayer;
listen to the words of my mouth.

For proud people have risen against me,
ruthless people seek my life.
They have no regard for God.
But I have God for my help.
The Lord upholds my life.

I will sacrifice to you with willing heart
and praise your name for it is good.
For you have rescued me from all my distress
and my eyes have seen the downfall of my foes.

FORGIVENESS AND HEALING
Cure of a Paralytic

Jesus got back in the boat, crossed the water and came to his own town. Then some people appeared, bringing him a paralytic stretched out on a bed. Seeing their faith, Jesus said to the paralytic: 'Courage, my child, your sins are forgiven'. And at this some of the scribes said to themselves: 'This man is blaspheming'. Knowing what was in their minds, Jesus said: 'Why do you have such wicked thoughts in your hearts? Now, which of these is easier to say, "Your sins are forgiven", or to say "Get up and walk"?' But to prove to you that the Son of Man has authority on earth to forgive sins — he said to the paralytic — 'Get up and pick up your bed and go off home'. And the man got up and went home. A feeling of awe came over the crowd when they saw this, and they praised God for giving such power to people. (Mt. 9, 1-8)

Reflection Sometimes people see illness as some kind of punishment from God for sins committed. This can be seen in how often people say things like: 'Why did this happen to me? I haven't done any harm to anyone.' A story like this one from St Matthew's Gospel would seem to confirm that belief where Jesus seems to link this man's disease with his sins; however this perception is false. God does not treat us like that. We believe that suffering results from Original Sin when humanity, in the figures of Adam and Eve, chose to go its own way rather than follow God's way to full life. The direction of human life changed utterly from that time.

This story is about something different. It is first of all a statement that Jesus, who has the power to heal, has an even greater power that touches an even more important need in every human life, namely to forgive us our sins and restore us to full communion with God. When we are ill our horizons get limited to our pain and suffering and our hopes get confined to being free from whatever is troubling us. The reality is that many people who are not suffering any physical pain are still deeply unhappy and the source of their unhappiness is the same as that of someone who is suffering. We all need forgiveness so that our hearts and souls can be at peace. Then we can face anything.

The second facet of this story worth noting is how limited the religious people's perception of God is. They believe they have God under their control and when Jesus does something that is not under that they condemn him. That is something that is common to many of us. But God is much larger than we imagine, so much so that he holds each of us in his heart as if we were his only child and loves us dearly. Intimacy with God is what Jesus offers and through that we will be healed.

Prayer God of all-embracing love, praise and glory to you for the many ways you show your love in my life. Send your Holy Spirit into my heart so that I may accept your gifts of forgiveness and healing, that my whole being may sing your praises and that all around me may know the wonders of your love. Take away from me all guilt, anxiety and fear so that I can bask in the knowledge of you and rest in your loving arms. I ask this in the name of Jesus your beloved Son. Amen.

Psalm 56

Have mercy on me God, have mercy
for in you my soul has taken refuge
in the shadow of your wings I take refuge
till the storms of destruction pass by.

I call to God the Most High
to God who has always been my help.
May he send from heaven and save me
and shame those who assail me.
May God send his truth and his love.

My heart is ready, O God,
my heart is ready.
I will sing, I will sing your praise.
Awake, my soul,
awake lyre and harp,
I will awake the dawn.

I thank you, Lord among the peoples,
among the nations I will praise you
for your love reaches to the heavens
and your truth to the skies.

O God, arise above the heavens;
may your glory shine on earth.

NO ILLNESS TOO BIG OR SMALL
Cure of Peter's Mother-In-Law

Going into Peter's house Jesus found Peter's mother-in-law in bed with fever. He touched her hand and the fever left her, and she got up and began to wait on him. (Mt. 8, 4)

Reflection There is no illness too big, or too small, for the power of Jesus to enter in and bring healing and hope. That is the clear message of the Gospel stories of healing. In this particular story we hear of Peter's mother-in-law with a fever. We might think of this as a rather minor illness, but it was significant to her in that she was unable to look after her family as a result.

Sometimes when we compare our own illnesses with those of others we gain a sense of proportion. But we can also think that it is not worth anyone's notice. The reality is that even a simple toothache, or a fever, or a sore head can cause pain and anxiety and may immobilise us. In these, as with more serious illnesses, we should take appropriate action to seek out medical help. But we also have the right to seek the help of Jesus who wants to be with us and speak his love to our hearts at these times of pain and doubt.

Prayer Lord Jesus, you entered into the home of Peter and brought healing. Come into our home and live with us. May we know the gentleness of your presence and the strength of your power. Help us to turn to you in all our needs and to praise you in all our joys. And when we are in pain help us never to despair, but to trust in your love and to place ourselves in your hands. Amen.

Psalm 22

The Lord is my shepherd;
there is nothing I shall want,
fresh and green are the pastures
where he gives me repose.
Near restful waters he leads me
to revive my drooping spirit.

He guides me along the right path;
He is true to his name.
If I should walk in the valley of darkness
no evil would I fear.
You are there with your crook and your staff;
with these you give me comfort.

You have prepared a banquet for me
in the sight of my foes
My head you have anointed with oil
my cup is overflowing.

Surely goodness and kindness shall follow me
all the days of my life.
In the Lord's own house shall I dwell
for ever and ever.

'I WILL COME MYSELF AND CURE HIM'
Cure of the Centurion's Servant

When he went into Capernaum a centurion came up and pleaded with him. 'Sir', he said, 'my servant is lying at home paralysed and in great pain.' 'I will come myself and cure him' said Jesus. The centurion replied, 'Sir, I am not worthy to have you under my roof; just give the word and my servant will be cured. For I am under authority myself, and have soldiers under me; and I say to one man: go and he goes; to another: come here and he comes; to my servant: do this, and he does it'. When Jesus heard this he was astonished and said to those following him, 'I tell you solemnly, nowhere in Israel have I found faith like this. And I tell you that many will come from east and west to take their places with Abraham and Isaac and Jacob at the feast in the kingdom of heaven; but the subjects of the kingdom will be turned out into the dark, where there will be weeping and grinding of teeth.' And to the centurion Jesus said, 'Go back then; you have believed, so let this be done for you.' And the servant was cured at that moment. (Mt. 8, 5-13)

Reflection Just before receiving Holy Communion we say: 'Lord, I am not worthy to receive you; only say the word and I shall be healed'. This is obviously taken from the story of the curing of the centurion's servant because there is such a similarity between that person and us. We are in need, especially when we are sick or when someone we love is sick. Jesus is always ready to come to us and to bring us healing. The most wonderful way he comes to us is in the Eucharist when he feeds us with his own Body and Blood. In most parishes today those who are sick can have Communion brought to them regularly. In hospitals there are people who are available to bring Communion daily. Think about availing of this wonderful gift that can bring you strength and comfort and will bring healing of body and spirit.

Prayer Even if you cannot receive Communion regularly you can think of the presence of Christ as very close to you and make a spiritual communion with him. This is a quiet prayer of longing for Him to be with you, knowing that this is His wish also.

Jesus, I believe that you are truly present in the Blessed Sacrament. I love you above all things and I desire you in my soul. As I cannot now receive you sacramentally, come at least spiritually into my heart. I unite myself entirely to you. Do not let me ever leave you.

O Sacrament most Holy, O Sacrament Divine, all praise and all thanksgiving be every moment Thine.

Psalm 76

I cry aloud to God
cry aloud to God that he may hear me.

In the day of my distress I sought the Lord.
My hands were raised at night without ceasing.
My soul refused to be consoled.
I remembered my God and I groaned.
I pondered and my spirit fainted.

You withheld sleep from my eyes
I was troubled, I could not speak.
I thought of the days of long ago
and remembered the years long past.
At night I mused within my heart
I pondered and my spirit questioned.

Your ways, O God, are holy.
What god is great as our God?
You are the God who works wonders.
You showed your power among the peoples.
Your strong arm redeemed your people,
the children of Jacob and Joseph.

FACING SUICIDE
Cure of the Man Born Blind

As Jesus went along, he saw a man who had been blind from birth. His disciple asked him, 'Rabbi, who sinned, this man or his parents, for him to have been born blind?' 'Neither he nor his parents sinned.' Jesus answered, 'he was born blind so that the works of God might be displayed in him.'

Having said this, he spat on the ground, made a paste with the spittle, put this over the eyes of the blind man and said to him, 'Go and wash in the Pool of Siloam' (a name which means 'sent'). So the blind man went off and washed himself, and came away with his sight restored. (Jn. 9, 1-3; 6-7)

Reflection One of the most alarming things happening in our society today is the number of people, especially young people who, blinded by despair or anxiety or fear, are taking their lives through suicide. One of the most common things that happens as a result is people being destroyed by guilt and apportioning blame. Parents especially look at themselves and wonder where they went wrong. Even if they can find no particular reason to blame themselves they still do. It is very like the reaction above: 'Who sinned, this person or her/his parents that this thing has happened?'

First of all we need to think of those who have taken this drastic step and pray for them that, whatever the reason, they will now be at peace with God. And we pray for their parents and families that God may be with them in very visible forms through good support and through prayer.

Secondly we need to think of those who may be tempted to go in this direction that we can find all the ways necessary to help them move away from the brink and find the goodness of life. The responsibility is a common one that involves the State, the Church, the schools, parents and the parish. Every resource possible is called for to help our young people today to have a real sense of the goodness of life and its wonderful possibilities. We will not provide those resources unless we are being led by the love of God.

Prayer Lord Jesus Christ, you are the Son of God and the Son of Mary. We ask you to be with us in the tragedies of human life, especially in the devastating phenomenon of suicide. Draw all those who have gone in this direction into your loving embrace and let them know the extent of your love. Bless the parents and families and friends of those who have committed suicide and help them to let go of their guilt and the blaming of themselves or others so that they may live in your peace and be able to hold their loved one in their hearts with affection.

Give us leaders in Church and State who will commit themselves to getting our society beyond the point where anyone would even think of taking her/his own life. May the values of human life which you brought to us, the values of love, take new root among us so that everyone can be treasured and where no one will ever have to go through life without the knowledge of your presence and your love. Amen.

Psalm 130

O Lord, my heart is not proud
nor haughty my eyes.
I have not gone after things too great
nor marvels beyond me.

Truly I have set my soul
in silence and peace.
As a child has rest in its mother's arms,
even so my soul.

O Israel, hope in the Lord
both now and forever.

RESTORING HUMAN DIGNITY
Cure of the Man with a Withered Hand

Jesus went again into a synagogue, and there was a man there who had a withered hand. And they were watching him to see if he would cure him on the Sabbath day, hoping for something to use against him. He said to the man with the withered hand: 'Stand out in the middle'. Then he said to them: 'Is it against the law on the Sabbath day to do good or to do evil; to save life, or to kill?' But they said nothing. Then, grieved to see them so obstinate, he looked angrily around at them, and said to the man: 'Stretch out your hand'. He stretched it out and his hand was better. The Pharisees went out and at once began to plot with the Herodians against him, discussing how to destroy him. (Mk. 3, 1-6)

Reflection There are several important things in this story to reflect on when we pray for healing. The first one is the power of prejudice in human life. The man had a withered hand – and there probably were people there who despised him because of that. We so easily judge one another by appearances and we live our lives by those judgements. That is not the way of Christ, so we need healing from that.

The second thing that stands out in the story is the attitude of the Pharisees. They were religious people who were gathered for their service, but what were they doing? They were watching Jesus to see if they could catch him out. We often need guidance for the ways we use religion to cover up our real attitudes to life. It's not just that our minds wander when we are praying, but rather that we use prayer as a ritual rather than as an action of the heart. Jesus was angry with them for being so obstinate because they did not see how much they needed his healing touch.

And thirdly there is this man who was in need of healing both of his hand and of his dignity. Jesus did not for a moment take his eyes off him because he loved him and wanted only what was good for him, even if that meant that he himself was put in danger. Through the power of the word that Jesus spoke in love this man's hand was healed. That is how Jesus is with each of us.

Prayer Jesus, we thank you and praise you for your love for each one of us. Through your spirit in us heal us from all prejudice so that we can bring dignity to every person we meet. Through that same spirit take away anything that makes our hearts hardened against anyone so that we may see each person as you see them. And be with us through your word and your love so that in our illness our bodies may be healed. Amen.

Psalm 17

I love you, Lord, my strength
my rock, my fortress, my saviour.
My God is the rock where I take refuge;
my shield, my mighty help, my stronghold.
The Lord is worthy of all praise:
when I call I am saved from my foes.

In my anguish I called to the Lord
I cried to my God for help.
From his temple he heard my voice,
my cry came to his ears.

You, O Lord, are my lamp,
my God who lightens my darkness.
With you I can break through any barrier,
with my God I can scale any wall.

Healing Blindness of Spirit
Cure of Two Blind Men

As Jesus went on his way two blind men followed him shouting, 'Take pity on us, Son of David'. And when Jesus reached the house the blind men came up with him and he said to them, 'Do you believe I can do this?' They said, 'Sir, we do'. Then he touched their eyes saying, 'Your faith deserves it, so let this be done for you'. And their sight returned. Then Jesus sternly warned them, 'Take care that no one learns about this'. But when they had gone, they talked about him all over the countryside. (Mt. 9, 27-31)

Reflection Every illness is difficult to cope with but blindness must be a particularly difficult cross to carry. It is hard to imagine living in darkness and not being able to see the beauty of the world in which we live or even the very ordinary things of everyday life. However there is an even worse blindness than physical loss of sight and that is the blindness of the spirit that very many suffer from.

This blindness of the spirit is caused in many people by becoming so busy that they don't have time to see the beauty of the world or even the wonder of the ordinary things of life. They are so concerned with getting ahead, but have no idea what the future holds so often end up in disappointment. Other people suffer from blindness of spirit because of their need to put themselves and their needs first; they cannot enjoy the company of loved ones and have no idea of the pleasure of serving people in need. Of course illnesses of all kinds cause blindness of spirit as they draw us into their own world of self-obsession, a world in which there is little room for gladness or joy or peace.

Jesus stands with us always and offers us healing that will lift us out of our small worlds of self-interest, self-involvement or of general selfishness and into the wonderful world of God's love where we can see clearly the beauty of His presence with us.

Prayer 'Take pity on us, Son of David' was the cry of the men who approached you in their need and their blindness. Jesus, we make that our cry also as we open ourselves up to your healing power. Be with us in our illness. Be with us also in our blindness of spirit so that we may see the goodness that is within us and all around us and so give glory to God from a heart set free by your love. We pray especially for those who are physically blind. Let them know your presence with them. And give all of us an awareness of how they need our help and an openness to learn from them how to see. Amen.

Psalm 61

In God alone is my soul at rest,
my help comes from him.
He alone is my rock, my stronghold,
my fortress, I stand firm.

In God is my safety and glory,
the rock of my strength.
Take refuge in God all you people.
Trust him at all times.
Pour out your hearts before him
for God is our refuge.

For God has said only one thing
only two do I know:
that to God alone belongs power
and to you, Lord, love
and that you repay each of us
according to our deeds.

GO IN PEACE

Cure of the Woman with a Haemorrhage

Now there was a woman suffering from a haemorrhage for twelve years whom no one had been able to cure. She came up behind Jesus and touched the fringe of his cloak; and the haemorrhage stopped at that instant. Jesus said, 'Who touched me?' When they all denied that they had, Peter and his companions said, 'Master, it is the crowds round you, pushing'. But Jesus said, 'Somebody touched me, I felt that power had gone out from me.' Seeing herself discovered, the woman came forward trembling, and falling at his feet explained in front of all the people why she had touched him and how she had been cured at that very moment. 'My daughter', he said, 'your faith has restored you to health; go in peace'. (Lk. 8, 43-48)

Reflection A lot of people, because of embarrassment or self-consciousness, neglect taking proper steps to see about their health. This is particularly true of men. They often find it hard to go to the doctor, and even when they do they often don't tell the entire truth about themselves. This can be because of the nature of their illness or because of the location of their problem. If you have this difficulty ask the Lord to help you overcome it and see to yourself immediately.

Other people can have a difficulty in approaching Christ for his help in their illness because of guilt or shame about their lifestyle or because they are conscious of not having been in touch with him for a long time. They can think of themselves as hypocrites in coming to him now when they are in serious need. Christ certainly does not want you to stay away from him because of this. We do not have to be good or religious to have immediate contact with him. The woman in this story is a great model for all of us of how Christ welcomes everyone who needs his help. He brings attention to her, not to put her on the spot, but to encourage all of us to reach out to him and let him speak his love to our hearts. How wonderful it is to hear him speak that word to us: 'Your faith has restored you to health. Go in peace.'

Prayer Lord Jesus Christ, you know our minds and hearts and you care about all our needs. Be with anyone who is finding it difficult to understand themselves because of embarrassment or self-consciousness. Help them to move beyond these inhibitions so that they can find the ways of approaching their doctor in time for the sake of their health. Bless anyone who finds it difficult to approach you because of anything in their lives of which they are ashamed or guilty. Help all of us to know the extent of your unconditional love, so that we can hear your word of healing spoken into our hearts. Amen.

Psalm 62

O God, you are my God, for you I long,
for you my soul is thirsting.
My body pines for you
like a dry, weary land without water.
So I gaze on you in the sanctuary
to see your strength and your glory.

For your love is better than life,
my lips will speak your praise.
So I will bless you all my life,
in your name I will lift up my hands.
My soul shall be filled as with a banquet
my mouth shall praise you with joy.

On my bed I remember you.
On you I muse through the night
for you have been my help;
in the shadow of your wings I rejoice.
My soul clings to you
your right hand holds me fast.

CARING FOR AN ALZHEIMER SUFFERER

Cures at Gennesaret

Having made the crossing, they came to land at Gennesaret. When the local people recognised Jesus they spread the news through the whole neighbourhood and took all who were sick to him, begging him just to let them touch the hem of his cloak. And all those who touched it were completely cured.

Reflection Illness doesn't just affect the person who is suffering from it. It affects those who are in close contact with the person either because of family or friendship ties or because of medical care. This is particularly true of an illness like Alzheimer disease. This is a relatively new phenomenon in human life. The person who suffers from it very often seems unaware of what is happening and can remain healthy in every other way. But for families it is often a source of great heartbreak. Their loved one – a wife/husband, mother/father – is no longer there and it is impossible to get in touch with her/him. There are all the feelings of loss. It is like a bereavement, but the person is still there in body.

As this can be a fairly long-term illness, other feelings are often very strong; feelings associated with bereavement. There is anger at the person for being like this. There is anger at God for leaving them in this state. There is anger at life for such a bad deal. And there can be family divisions caused by all of this. It is not a pleasant place to be for any of us.

We can bring those with Alzheimer disease to Jesus and ask him to bless them and be with them in their isolation. But we should also bring those who love them to him and ask him to heal them in all the ways they need his healing power – to help them to continue to reverence their loved one who has the disease; to give them peace within themselves and patience with others; to strengthen them for the days and weeks and months and even years that they have to carry this cross of heartbreak.

Prayer God our Creator, we thank you for all the gifts of life. We thank you for the wonder of our human minds especially, through which we can think and know and remember. Be with all those who have lost this wonderful gift in their lives and comfort them in their isolation. We pray especially for those who care for them. We pray for their families that you will be with them in the heartbreak of losing their loved one in this way. Strengthen them for the long road of grieving. Give them patience with themselves and one another. And give them your gift of peace so that they may be able to continue to reverence their loved one throughout this illness. Be with those responsible for medical care of all our sick, but especially those who have lost their ability to think or to remember so that they will always treat those in their care with reverence. Amen.

Psalm 118

My soul lies down in the dust;
by your word revive me.
I declared your ways and you answered
teach me your statutes.

Make me grasp the way of your precepts
and I will muse on your wonders.
My soul pines away with grief;
by your word raise me up.

Keep me from the way of error
and teach me your law.
I have chosen the way of truth
with your decrees before me.
I bind myself to do your will;
Lord, do not disappoint me.
I will run the way of your commands;
you give freedom to my heart.

TIMES OF DEPRESSION
Cures Near the Lake

Jesus went on from there and reached the shores of the lake of Galilee, and he went up into the hills. He sat there, and large crowds came to him bringing the lame, the crippled, the blind, the dumb and many others; these they put down at his feet, and he cured them. The crowds were astonished to see the dumb speaking, the cripples whole again, the lame walking and the blind with their sight, and they praised the God of Israel. (Mt. 15, 29-31)

Reflection There are so many things that go wrong with the human condition and yet life for most of us is good. However, there is one condition in which life does not seem good at any level and that is the condition of depression. It is a horrific disease to have for many reasons. First of all it is a very dark place to be and only those who have been there can know what it is like. It is a place where hope is most often missing and the future seems very bleak. Secondly, unlike a physical disease, others find it difficult to have sympathy for a person who is depressed and tend to avoid her or him when possible. Thirdly, people with depression often neglect the medication or the therapy that will help them get better and so the disease gets worse and the hopelessness deepens.

If you suffer from depression, don't lose heart. There is help for you in medicine and in good therapy. There are also groups around who can help you live with this disease and work your way towards health. And there is the power of Jesus available to you, a power that is not meant to take the place of the medical help that you need, but rather to give you the strength and confidence to seek out that help and to follow it. Through the power of Jesus the lame walked again, the blind had their sight restored, the dumb spoke again. Through that same power you too will find your way out of the darkness into the light of hope and joy.

Prayer Lord Jesus Christ, for the three days you lay dead in the tomb, we ask you to be with and bless all those who are suffering from depression or any other form of mental or emotional illness. Let them know your presence even in the darkness of their lives. And through knowing your presence give them hope and the confidence to look for and accept the help they need to move towards the light. We pray also for all those who are associated in any way with these, our sisters and brothers, either as carers or as family members or friends. Enrich them with compassion and with patience. Help them to understand more fully the agony of being locked into an inner world so that through their help and love those who are sick may be encouraged and helped towards health and well-being. Amen.

Psalm 5

To my words give ear, O Lord,
give heed to my groaning.
Attend to the sound of my cries
my King and my God.

It is you whom I invoke, O Lord.
In the morning you hear me;
in the morning I offer you my prayer
watching and waiting.

You are no God who loves evil;
no sinner is your guest.
The boastful shall not stand their ground
before your face.

But I through the greatness of your love
have access to your house.
I bow down before your holy temple
filled with awe.

All those you protect shall be glad
and ring out their joy.
You shelter them; in you they rejoice,
those who love your name.

PRAYING FOR A CHILD IN THE WOMB
Healing of a Cripple

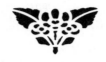

A man sat there who had never walked in his life, because his feet were crippled from birth; and as he listened to Paul preaching, he managed to catch his eye. Seeing that the man had the faith to be cured, Paul said in a loud voice, 'Get to your feet — stand up', and the cripple jumped up and began to walk. (Acts 14, 10)

Reflection In this story, as in all the stories of the Scriptures, we are in touch with much more than one person. This man who was born crippled is a symbol of the human condition just as Paul is a symbol of the desire and the power of our loving God. All kinds of things happen to the human person in the womb and at birth, which contribute to the struggle of life for each one. Very many people are born crippled in one way or another and will need that touch of God through their lives if they are ever to 'jump up and begin to walk'.

When a child is conceived, a lot is already determined about her or his future because of the genes of the parents. Other things become determined over the next nine months as the child grows in the womb because of the positive or negative behaviour of the parents. It is a fairly normal reaction to the news of pregnancy that parents are shocked or surprised or even rejecting of the baby that has been conceived. If this lasts through the nine months the baby will be greatly affected by it. Research shows that a mother who smokes during pregnancy can be putting the child at risk and the same is true of the use of alcohol. But it is not only the mother's responsibility to prepare for the birth of the child in every way that is possible so that the baby will be welcomed with warmth and affection. This is also the task of the father and of all those who will be involved with that child's life as she/he grows to maturity.

We need to call on God's power to bring the child in the womb to a safe birth and a fulfilled life. The parents of the unborn child can pray for and bless their baby every day and so grow in an awareness of and love for their little one. All of us have a responsibility to ensure the well-being of the next generation and one of the ways we can effectively do this is by praying regularly for those who are preparing to enter this world of ours.

Prayer · *Parents* God, co-creator with us of our child in this womb, we thank you for the wonders of your love for us. Bless our new baby and keep her or him safe from all harm as she or he prepares for entry into our family life and the world in which we live. Be with us as parents that we may have the generosity and the courage to do all that is necessary to make this home a place of love and affection so that our baby may know now that it is a good place to be. Over the weeks or months ahead may we do everything in our power to keep this new life safe. Through your Spirit speak into the heart of our little one the words we speak: 'We love you'. Amen.

Others Creator God, we thank you for entrusting us with the power to create with you the new life of our children. We pray for all unborn children that they may be loved and cherished by their parents and kept safe from all harm. We pray for the parents of unborn children that they may have generosity of love for each other so that their child may enter into a world of warmth and affection. Bless all parents who have lost a child through miscarriage. Help them to know that their little one is with you and still part of their lives. Bless all parents who have lost a child through abortion. Help them to accept the forgiveness of their little one as they accept your forgiveness and love. We make our prayer through Christ our Lord. Amen.

Psalm 138

It was you who created my being
knit me together in my mother's womb.
I thank you for the wonder of my being,
for the wonders of all your creation.

Already you knew my soul,
my body held no secret from you
when I was being fashioned in secret
and moulded in the depths of the earth.

Your eyes saw all my actions,
they were all of them written in your book.
Every one of my days was decreed
before one of them came into being.

To me how mysterious your thoughts,
the sum of them not to be numbered.
If I count them, they are more than the sand;
to finish, I must be eternal like you.

O search me, God, and know my heart.
O test me and know my thoughts.
See that I follow not the wrong path
and lead me in the path of life eternal.

EMBARRASSING ILLNESSES
Healing of a Dropsical Man on the Sabbath

Now on a Sabbath day Jesus had gone for a meal to the house of one of the leading Pharisees; and they watched him closely. There in front of him was a man with dropsy, and Jesus addressed the lawyers and Pharisees. 'Is it against the law', he asked, 'to cure a man on the Sabbath, or not?' But they remained silent, so he took the man and cured him and sent him away. Then he said to them, 'Which of you here, if his son falls into a well, or his ox, will not pull him out on a Sabbath day without hesitation?' And to this they could find no answer. (Lk. 14, 1-5)

Reflection The dictionary defines dropsy as: 'a disease causing watery fluid to collect in the body.' It must be a very distressing disease as well as a very embarrassing one. Of course there is medication for this kind of disease today, which did not exist in the time of Jesus, and anyone who suffers from this should seek out help.

Unfortunately, someone with a disease like this is often the object of ridicule from others. And this is one of the points in the story of the Gospel. In almost every story of healing either other people or the sick person asks Jesus for healing. No one has any pity for this man; they take no notice of him. And he sees himself as of no value either. In this instance Jesus takes the initiative and heals him. It is a direct challenge to the hard-hearted attitudes of these religious people. And it is a direct statement of how Jesus values every person no matter what his or her appearance or status.

In this we find two of the ways we all need the healing power of Jesus. We need him to free us from the prejudices we hold towards others who do not measure up to the false standards of respect that we set for ourselves in society. There is so much pain and suffering caused by how we treat people who do not look or sound the way we expect. And we need Jesus to help us rejoice in our own human dignity no matter what is happening to us in our own life. It doesn't matter if we are tall or short, heavy or light, old or young, male or female. All that matters is that each person is equally made in the image of God and loved by God and has a right to be loved and respected by us; that is true religion.

Prayer Loving God, through your Son Jesus Christ, you assure us that you are one who loves each of us as we are. Through the power of your Spirit, help us to believe this about ourselves and about everyone we meet and to live out this belief in our lives. Forgive us for the ways we have harmed others through our prejudices and help us to repent for that. Send your Spirit into the depths of our society so that everyone may receive the reverence and respect that is our right as your daughters and sons. Help us to rid our minds and hearts and our society of the evil of bullying, which is always based on the perceived weakness of those being bullied, so that we can live in peace with one another and with hope shining out in our lives. Amen.

Psalm 45

God is for us a refuge and strength,
a helper close at hand, in time of distress.
So we shall not fear though the earth should rock,
though the mountains fall into the depths of the sea,
even though its waters rage and foam,
even though the mountains be shaken by its waves.

The waters of a river give joy to God's city,
the holy place where the Most High dwells.
God is within, it cannot be shaken;
God will help it at the dawning of the day.
Nations are in tumult, kingdoms are shaken;
he lifts his voice, the earth shrinks away.
Come, consider the works of the Lord
the redoubtable deeds he has done on the earth.
He puts an end to wars over all the earth;
the bow he breaks, the spear he snaps.
He burns the shields with fire.
'Be still and know that I am God,
supreme among the nations, supreme on the earth.'

The Lord of hosts is with us;
the God of Jacob is our stronghold.

COPING WITH DISABILITIES
Healing of a Deaf Man

Returning from the district of Tyre, he went by way of Sidon towards the Sea of Galilee, right through the Decapolis region. And they brought him a deaf man who had an impediment in his speech; and they asked him to lay his hands on him. He took him aside in private, away from the crowd, put his fingers into the man's ears and touched his tongue with spittle. Then looking up to heaven he sighed; and he said to him, 'Ephphatha', that is, 'Be opened'. And his ears were opened, and the ligament of his tongue was loosened and he spoke clearly. And Jesus ordered them to tell no one about it, but the more he insisted, the more widely they published it. Their admiration was unbounded. 'He has done all things well', they said, 'he makes the deaf hear and the dumb speak.' (Mk .7, 31-37)

Reflection In the summer of 2003 Ireland had the privilege of hosting the Special Olympics. Athletes with a variety of disabilities flocked here from every part of the world, along with their families and friends. Cities, towns and villages all over the country hosted these special guests. The whole country hummed with excitement and with the quiet joy of a people who knew that God was visiting his people in an extraordinary way.

The special athletes taught us that disability, far from making a person less human, can in many ways make her or him more human. Their parents who came among us taught us the generosity of love that made them treasure these children of theirs. And their coaches and other training personnel taught us to believe in every person's gifts and not be distracted by what is perceived as human blemish. The thousands of volunteers who gave their time and energy so generously taught us that Irish people are not totally committed to the worship of the Celtic Tiger.

In a very real way, the ears of a whole nation were opened to hear the good news of what being truly human is and their tongues were loosened to rejoice in what is essential to human living. This miracle has to be kept alive in us as we grow to treasure every person and demand that all the resources of Church and State be put at the service of those with disabilities. It is they who can best keep us fully human.

Prayer Lord Jesus Christ, with love you put your fingers into the ears of the deaf man and put your spittle on his tongue and so restored him to full life. We pray for ourselves that we can experience that same love you have for each one of us in the ways we need you in our own lives. We pray for healing for our society that we can become ever more a people that treasures every individual person. Bring us to generosity in caring for one another. And open our hearts to learn from those whom the world seeks to reject. Bless all parents of children with disabilities. Keep them steadfast in their love. And help us to support them in every way they need. Especially we ask that you would give us the courage to insist that our governments would invest heavily in caring for those who can so easily be neglected so that our world can ring out with gladness and joy in your love and your presence. Amen.

Psalm 116

O praise the Lord, all you nations
acclaim him all you peoples!

Strong is his love for us
he is faithful forever.

Glory be to the Father and to the Son and to the Holy Spirit
as it was in the beginning, is now and ever shall be
world without end. Amen.

HEALING FROM SEXISM
Healing of a Crippled Woman on the Sabbath

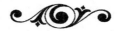

One Sabbath day Jesus was teaching in one of the synagogues and a woman was there who for eighteen years had been possessed by a spirit that left her enfeebled; she was bent double and quite unable to stand upright. When Jesus saw her he called her over and said, 'Woman, you are rid of your infirmity' and he laid his hands on her. And at once she straightened up, and she glorified God.

But the synagogue official was indignant because Jesus had healed on the Sabbath and he addressed the people present. 'There are six days', he said, 'when work is to be done. Come and be healed on one of those days and not on the Sabbath'. But the Lord answered him. 'Hypocrites!' he said. (Lk. 13, 10-15)

Reflection A very special feature of the Gospels is the way Jesus deals with women. Many cultures regarded women as inferior to men or as the possession of men. Jesus treated women as equal and dealt with them with great love and tenderness. He included women among his disciples, much to the horror of the religious leaders of his time.

Unfortunately, the Church has adapted the Gospel to the culture of society on this as on many other issues. The demon of sexism has kept women in bondage in the Church as in society for generations. Terrible damage has been done to human dignity because of this. And attempts are constantly made to justify it because of the law. We need to pray for a change of heart in the Church and a deep healing in the lives of those who have been damaged either as victims of this mentality or as the perpetrators of it. The Church owes a great debt of gratitude to the women who have been faithful through all of this. We now owe women a full say in how they see themselves as part of the Body of Christ to the glory of God. The contrast between Jesus and the synagogue official in the story above is constantly being played out among us. Our task is to make sure that the healing touch of Jesus always wins out over the hardness of heart of the official.

Prayer Lord Jesus Christ, you reveal to us the True God, a God of love and compassion and a God who is passionate in his love for us. You also reveal to us our true humanity in all its fullness. Forgive us for the ways we set limits to your revelation and settle for our own images and our own idols. Through your Spirit living in us heal the evil of sexism in our Church so that we can be a witness to the society in which we live. Help us to acknowledge our equality with one another and face all the implications of that so that your people may be healed and your Spirit may be set free. Bless all women and reward them for their tremendous faithfulness to the Church through the generations. May we have the ability to work together for the transformation of our world into your kingdom of peace and love. Amen.

Psalm 113B

Not to us, Lord, not to us,
but to your name give the glory
for the sake of your love and your truth,
lest the heathen say: 'where is their God?'

But our God is in the heavens;
he does whatever he wills.
Their idols are silver and gold,
the work of human hands.

They have mouths but they cannot speak;
they have eyes but they cannot see;
they have ears but they cannot hear;
they have nostrils but they cannot smell.

The Lord will bless those who fear him,
the little no less than the great.
To you may the Lord grant increase,
to you and all your children.

We who live bless the Lord
now and forever. Amen.

CARING FOR CARERS
Jairus' Daughter Raised to Life

On his return Jesus was welcomed by the crowd, for they were all waiting for him. And now there came a man named Jairus, who was an official of the synagogue. He fell at Jesus' feet and pleaded with him to come to his house because he had a daughter about twelve years old, who was dying. And the crowds were almost stifling Jesus as he went.

While he was still speaking, someone came from the house of the synagogue official to say, 'Your daughter has died. Do not trouble the Master any further'. But Jesus heard this, and he spoke to the man, 'Do not be afraid, only have faith and she will be safe'. When he came to the house he allowed no one to go in with him except Peter and John and James, and the child's father and mother. They were all weeping and mourning for her, but Jesus said, 'Stop crying; she is not dead, but asleep'. But they laughed at him, knowing she was dead. But taking her by the hand he called to her, 'Child, get up'. And her spirit returned and she got up at once. Then he told them to give her something to eat. Her parents were astonished, but he ordered them not to tell anyone what had happened. (Lk. 8, 40-42; 48-56)

Reflection This story highlights many wonderful qualities of Jesus that are important for us to keep in mind. Firstly, he is equally at ease with a crowd as with individuals. In fact in the midst of the crowd he is fully aware of the individual. Secondly, he has a heartfelt compassion for the heartbreak of this father whose young daughter was dying. His compassion prompted him to leave the crowd immediately and go with Jairus. Thirdly, he has strength to face the laughter of those who were in the house so that this in no way put him off. Fourthly, he acknowledges the dignity of his disciples and the parents of the young girl as he brought them into the room with him. Fifthly, he has such gentleness as he speaks to the young girl, calling her back to life. And finally, he is so very practical as he tells them to give her something to eat. Those are also some of the qualities he demonstrates as he comes to us in our needs. All we have to do is call on him and let ourselves be carried along in his arms. We can know especially the beauty of his compassion, his personal love for each of us, and his gentleness as he speaks his healing word into our lives.

Prayer Lord Jesus Christ, help me to know more fully the extent of your love for me. As someone who cares for a loved one who is ill, I need your help every day. When I feel angry help me to be kind. When I feel used help me to be gentle. When I feel isolated help me to remember the isolation of the person I am caring for. When I feel tired help me to relax so that I don't take this out on the sick. When I feel self-pity help me to forget myself and concentrate my love on the person I care for. When I feel like giving up help me to have renewed strength. Amen.

Psalm 26

O Lord, hear my voice when I call,
have mercy and answer.
Of you my heart has spoken
'Seek his face.'

It is your face, O Lord, that I seek;
hide not your face.
Dismiss not your servant in anger;
you have been my help.

Do not abandon or forsake me,
O God my help.
Though father and mother forsake me,
the Lord will receive me.

I am sure I shall see the Lord's goodness
in the land of the living.
Hope in him, hold firm and take heart.
hope in the Lord.

RESTORING THE CHURCH COMMUNITY

Paul Raises a Dead Man to Life

On the first day of the week we met to break bread, Paul was due to leave the next day, and he preached a sermon that went on till the middle of the night. A number of lamps were lit in the upstairs room where we were assembled, and as Paul went on and on, a young man called Eutychus who was sitting on the windowsill grew drowsy and was overcome by sleep and fell to the ground three floors below. He was picked up dead. Paul went down and stooped to clasp the boy to him. 'There is no need to worry', he said, 'there is still life in him'. Then he went back upstairs where he broke bread and ate and carried on talking till he left at daybreak. They took the boy away alive, and were greatly encouraged. (Acts 20, 7-12)

Reflection There is a spiritual illness today that needs a lot of attention from all of us, namely the alienation from the life of the Church that has taken place for so many people because of the sins and sometimes the crimes of others. It is like a spiritual death, and many people are suffering greatly because of it. As with every illness, there is a lot of denial in us and we try to go on as if everything is normal. We need to face up to the terrible reality and repent of the sins that have been committed against some of the most vulnerable people among us. There is also so much anger because of these sins that a way

66

forward is so easily blocked. We need to find the ways of unblocking ourselves by easing the anger and eventually getting rid of it through reconciliation. Great mistakes have been made which need to be put right. This can lead to changes in the structures of the Church, changes that are resisted by people in positions of power. But they need to let go of their vested interests for the sake of the faith of our people and the salvation of Christ for our world.

Paul's words: 'Do not be afraid, there is still life in him' can give us confidence for going forward. There is still life in the Church. It just needs to be nurtured through prayer and penance. It also needs to be nurtured through taking care of each individual, both those who have been damaged and those who have done the damage. It is a time for each of us to exercise the core of our faith, namely that Christ is among us and nothing should ever become more important to us than that wonderful truth. And Christ among us can and will heal our wounds and bring us back to full life.

Prayer Lord Jesus Christ, you gather us to you in your Church so that each one may come to know the extent of your love and that the world may believe and so be saved. Forgive us for the many ways we are unfaithful to you. Heal the wounds of those among us who have been seriously damaged through abuse – physical, sexual, emotional, spiritual. Help us also to find the ways of ministering to those who have caused the abuse. Heal the wounds also for those who have been damaged through the abuse of power in the Church. We pray especially for healing and forgiveness for the ways that women have been and are treated as less than men among your people. Help us to restore confidence among our people in your presence and your love. And continue to shape us in your image so that the world may believe in you and so come to know our Father's love. Amen.

Psalm 118

Teach me the demands of your precepts
and I will keep them to the end.
Train me to observe your law,
to keep it with my heart.

Guide me in the path of your commands,
for there is my delight.
Bend my heart to your will
and not to love of gain.

Keep my eyes from what is false,
by your word give me life.
Keep the promise you have made
to the servant who fears you.

Keep me from the scorn I dread,
for your decrees are good.
See I long for your precepts;
then in your justice, give me life.

CARING FOR THOSE WHO ARE HOUSEBOUND

Peter Cures a Paralytic at Lydda

Peter visited one place after another and eventually came to the saints living down in Lydda. There he found a man called Aeneas, a paralytic who had been bedridden for eight years. Peter said to him, 'Aeneas, Jesus Christ cures you; get up and fold up your sleeping mat'. Aeneas got up immediately; everybody who lived in Lydda and Sharon saw him, and they were all converted to the Lord. (Acts 9, 32-35)

Reflection Many people have to carry the very heavy cross of being housebound or bedridden for a long period of time because of illness. The man Peter met in this story had been like this for eight years. Many people suffer even longer and there seems to be no relief for them.

The illness itself is a great cross, but it is complicated by immobility. A person loses their independence by having their actions overseen by a carer or having the carer effectively do everything for them. A person who is housebound or bedridden is like a captive audience for others with little or no say in what happens from day to day. It can be a time of great frustration that can lead to anger and no one, not even the person herself or himself, knows where the anger comes from. Misunderstandings can easily arise between the person who is ill and those who are looking after her/him.

It is also a very difficult time for the carers. They are deeply distressed by the fact that someone they love is so ill. They do their very best to take care of this loved one. But it seems to go on endlessly and at times they can also get frustrated and angry. They are ashamed of themselves for feeling like this and a vicious circle can be entered into between the carers and the person who is ill.

Peter always represents the people of the Church. This story is a call for the community to care for the housebound and those who are bedridden. He also seeks to assist those who are caring for them so that they may come through this difficult time with dignity and a knowledge of the presence of Christ.

Prayer Lord Jesus Christ, we thank you and praise you for the wonderful ways you are with us. Help us to know your presence each day. Be with those who are suffering long-term illness, especially those who have the cross of being housebound or bedridden as a result. Give them great peace of mind and heart. Help them to join their sufferings with your death on the Cross so that the cross they carry may be fruitful for the salvation of the world. Through your presence with them may they never lose heart. Be with those who care for these sisters and brothers of ours. Help them to be patient with themselves, especially at times when they feel frustrated or angry. Bring them safely through these times so that they can grow in their love for those they care for. And help us all, as the community of your Church, to take our place in bringing health and peace to those who need our help. Amen.

Psalm 15

Preserve me God, I take refuge in you.
I say to the Lord 'You are my God'.
My happiness lies in you alone.

O Lord, it is you who are my portion and cup,
it is you yourself who are my prize.
The lot marked out for me is my delight,
welcome indeed the heritage that falls to me.

I will bless the Lord who gives me counsel
who even at night directs my heart.
I keep the Lord ever in my sight.
Since he is at my right hand, I shall stand firm.
And so my heart rejoices, my soul is glad,
even my body shall rest in safety.
For you will not leave my soul among the dead,
nor let your beloved know decay.

You will show me the path of life
the fullness of joy in your presence,
at your right hand happiness forever.

COPING WITH GROWING OLD
Peter Raises a Woman to Life at Jaffa

At Jaffa there was a woman disciple called Tabitha, or Dorcas in Greek, who never tired of doing good or giving in charity. But the time came when she got ill and died, and they washed her and laid her out in a room upstairs. Lydda is not far from Jaffa, so when the disciples heard that Peter was there, they sent two men with an urgent message for him, 'Come and visit us as soon as possible'.

Peter went back with them straightaway, and on his arrival they took him to the upstairs room, where all the widows stood round in tears, showing him tunics and other clothes Dorcas had made when she was with them. Peter sent them all out of the room and knelt down and prayed. Then he turned to the dead woman and said, 'Tabitha, stand up'. She opened her eyes, looked at Peter and sat up. Peter helped her to her feet, then he called in the saints and widows and showed them she was alive. The whole of Jaffa heard about it and many believed in the Lord. (Acts 9, 36-42)

Reflection There is one condition of human life for which there is no cure, namely growing old. Of course it is not a disease, but it is a time when there can be many illnesses to cope with. Many people cope very well with old age, others find it extremely difficult. It is a time in life when we need to know the presence of Christ and find from him the gift of peace.

One of the very sad things that happens when a person grows old is that the community to which they belong and to whom many of them were very faithful over years can neglect them. The story above is a strong call to all of us today to take care of our elderly so that they can experience the tender care of Jesus working through us. Of course this has to begin with the families of the elderly. It may happen in our society that they are put into a nursing home and, while not forgotten, can be greatly neglected. Even those who are fortunate to continue to live in their own homes can spend days without ever speaking to another human being. We have a responsibility to make sure this does not happen. How we care for and reverence our elderly is a sign of how we care for and reverence Christ.

Prayer God of love, we thank you for the wonderful gift of human life made in your own image and likeness. We thank you for the adventure of all the stages of our lives from birth to old age to death and back to you. Help us to know your presence in our lives at each of the stages; especially the one each of us is in at this time so that we can be filled with your peace and gladness. We pray especially for those who are in old age just now. Be with them to comfort their hearts. Through your Spirit of love, help them to know that growing old is not just about coming towards the end of life, but also about coming towards the beginning of a new and even more wonderful adventure with you in eternity. Ease any burden of regret or guilt that anyone may have at this stage of life so that your peace and joy may be the qualities they are able to live with. Bless our families and faith communities with openness and generosity in caring for our elderly so that through us they may always know your presence and your love. We ask this through Christ our Lord. Amen.

Psalm 103

How many are your works, O Lord.
In wisdom you have made them all.
The earth is full of your riches.

All of them look to you
to give them their food in due season.
You give it, they gather it up;
you open your hand, they have their fill.

I will sing to the Lord all my life,
Make music to my God while I live.
May my thoughts be pleasing to him.
I find my joy in the Lord.
Let sinners vanish from the earth
and the wicked exist no more.

Bless the Lord, my soul.

FEELING ABANDONED
The Blind Man of Jericho

They reached Jericho; and as Jesus left Jericho with his disciples and a large crowd, Bartimaeus (that is, the son of Timaeus), a blind beggar, was sitting at the side of the road. When he heard it was Jesus of Nazareth, he began to shout and to say, 'Son of David, Jesus, have pity on me'. And many of them scolded him and told him to keep quiet, but he only shouted all the louder, 'Son of David, have pity on me'. Jesus stopped and said, 'Call him here'. So they called the blind man. 'Courage', they said 'get up; he is calling you.' So throwing off his cloak, he jumped up and went to Jesus. Then Jesus spoke, 'What do you want me to do for you?' 'Rabbi', the blind man said to him, 'Master, let me see again.' Jesus said to him, 'Go; your faith has saved you'. And immediately his sight returned and he followed him along the road. (Mk 10, 46-52)

Reflection One of the striking features of many of the stories of healing in the Gospels is that other people bring the sick to Jesus or bring him to them. In this story Bartimaeus is on his own and has to make his own way. Many people are like that and it can be a very difficult way to be. We see this in the lives of many of our elderly people who have no one to visit them or take care of them. Some of them are in their own homes and they see no one from one end of the day to the other. Others are in nursing homes and are left there by their families who very seldom visit them.

Illness is a time of aloneness by its very nature, but how difficult it is to have to bear it with little or no support.

It is out of this aloneness that Bartimaeus shouts out to Jesus: 'Son of David, Jesus, have pity on me.' Those who were closest to Jesus tried to silence him because they were missing the point of his presence. However, Jesus immediately reached out to him with the question: 'What do you want me to do for you?' And that is how he approaches each one of us. So don't hesitate to speak to him, telling him what you want him to do for you. You will not be disappointed. Those who are closest to Jesus in terms of listening to his word and in practice of faith need also to learn that he wants us to care for one another, with a special regard for those who are on their own.

Prayer Lord Jesus Christ, in your agony in the Garden you cried out: 'My God, my God, why have you abandoned me?' You know what it is like to be totally alone, with no one to care for you. Help me, when I reach the depths of loneliness, to know that you have been there before me and that, through your Spirit, I can meet you there. Help me not to despair but, even in the depths, that I may know the peace that you bring. Help me to reach out to others who may be in even greater need than I am so that I can bring your strength and consolation to them. And bring me to the next place you went in your agony: 'Not my will, but your will be done.' Amen.

Psalm 129

Out of the depths I cry to you, O Lord,
Lord hear my voice.
O let your ears be attentive
to the voice of my pleading.

If you, O Lord, should mark our guilt,
Lord, who would survive?
but with you is found forgiveness
For this we revere you.

My soul is waiting for the Lord,
I count on his word.
My soul is longing for the Lord
more than watchman for daybreak.
Let the watchman count on daybreak
and Israel on the Lord.

Because with the Lord there is mercy
and fullness of redemption.
Israel indeed he will redeem
from all its iniquity.

FACING NEW CHALLENGES
The Cure of a Lame Man

Once, when Peter and John were going up to the Temple for the prayers at the ninth hour, it happened that there was a man being carried past. He was a cripple from birth; and they used to put him down every day near the Temple entrance called the Beautiful Gate so that he could beg from the people going in. When this man saw Peter and John on their way into the Temple he begged from them. Both Peter and John looked straight at him and said, 'Look at us'. He turned to them expectantly, hoping to get something from them, but Peter said, 'I have neither silver nor gold, but I will give you what I have; in the name of Jesus Christ the Nazarene, walk.' Peter then took him by the hand and helped him to stand up. Instantly his feet and ankles became firm, he jumped up, stood, and began to walk, and he went with them into the Temple, walking and jumping and praising God. Everyone could see him walking and praising God and they recognised him as the man who used to sit begging at the Beautiful Gate of the Temple. They were all astonished and unable to explain what had happened to him. (Acts 3, 1-10)

Reflection One of the occupational hazards for the Church is to think that we have to have answers for all of life's problems so that we can solve them. There are many of these arising today from advances in science and technology and also in a greater sense of freedom that people are discovering and exercising. People are struggling with new issues of infertility. There are more public questions about sexual orientation. There are new and devastating diseases like HIV/AIDS. And at least some are looking to the Church for what we can offer in these life struggles. Of course we have to search out the moral and ethical responses to today's questions. But we also have to learn from this lovely story from the Acts of the Apostles. We may not have all the answers or solutions. But we do have what Peter and John offered; the name and the power of Jesus Christ.

What a wonderful gift we have to bring to every person and we should offer that gift with confidence and compassion and with the deepest humility. Together with Christ and with one another we can then find the way forward to a better world.

Prayer Lord Jesus Christ, we live in a world of great beauty and also of great confusion. We thank you for your presence with us in all of that. Help us, your Church, to seek answers to the many questions that trouble people today and to be faithful to your word in our searching. Help us also to have a real tenderness and compassion for each person as she or he is, so that no one will ever feel excluded from your presence and your love by the way we live or the way we teach and preach. Help us to know that the greatest gift we have for our world is you, our loving Lord and Saviour, and give us the confidence to let your love and your healing power be known to everyone. Amen.

Psalm 30

In you, O Lord, I take refuge.
Let me never be put to shame.
In your justice set me free,
hear me and speedily rescue me.

Be a rock of refuge for me,
a mighty stronghold to save me,
for you are my rock, my stronghold.
For your name's sake lead me and guide me.

Release me from the snares they have hidden
for you are my refuge, Lord.
Into your hands I commend my spirit,
it is you who will redeem me Lord.

O God of truth, you detest
those who worship false and empty gods.
As for me, I trust in the Lord.
Let me be glad and rejoice in your love.

Let your face shine on your servant.
Save me in your love.

LETTING GO TO CHRIST

The Cure of a Sick Man at the Pool of Bethzatha

Some time after this there was a Jewish festival, and Jesus went up to Jerusalem. Now, at the Sheep Pool in Jerusalem there is a building, called Bethzatha in Hebrew, consisting of five porticos; and under these were sick people – blind, lame, paralysed – waiting for the water to move; for at intervals the angel of the Lord came down into the pool, and the water was disturbed, and the first person to enter the water after this disturbance was cured of any ailment he or she suffered from. One man there had an illness which had lasted thirty-eight years, and when Jesus saw him lying there and knew he had been in this condition for a long time, he said, 'Do you want to be well again?' 'Sir', replied the sick man, 'I have no one to put me into the pool when the water is disturbed; and while I am still on the way, someone else gets there before me.' Jesus said: 'Get up, pick up your sleeping mat and walk'. The man was cured at once, and he picked up his mat and walked away. (Jn. 5, 1-9)

Reflection In this story we find the question that was chosen as the title of this book: 'Do you want to be well again?' It was asked of a man who had been ill for thirty-eight years. Wouldn't you expect someone like that to immediately say: 'Yes, of course, I want to be well again.' But that is not what happens. The first thing he says is: 'I have no one to put me into the pool when the waters are disturbed'. Because of his illness he had become so consumed with self-pity that he could not hear the offer that was being made. The second thing he says is: 'while I am still on the way someone else gets there before me'. Anger at those around him made him blame others for the fact that he was still in this condition. As a result of this he had more or less given up hope that he would ever know good health again. Those are the kind of reactions that are fairly normal in the presence of sickness, especially when this is on-going. It is precisely these reactions that Jesus wants to bring us through so that our hearts can find peace even in the midst of terrible suffering and that we can continue to have hope even when things seem completely hopeless.

Prayer Lord Jesus Christ, Son of the living God, open my mind and heart to know your presence with me so that I can hear your question and your offer of healing. When I am in danger of being overcome with self-pity or anger because of my illness, give me patience and peace. And when I am tempted to despair give me hope so that I may live each day to the full and that I may bring joy and gladness to all those who care for me and those whom I meet. Amen.

Psalm 39

I waited, I waited for the Lord
and he stooped down to me,
he heard my cry.

He drew me from the deadly pit,
from the miry clay.
He set my feet upon a rock
and made my footsteps firm.

He put a new song into my mouth
praise of our God.
Many shall see and fear
and shall trust in the Lord.

How many, O Lord my God
are the wonders and designs
that you have worked for us.
You have no equal.
Should I proclaim and speak of them
they are more than I can tell.

ACT OF SUBMISSION TO THE WILL OF GOD

My God, I do not know what will happen to me today. I only know that nothing will happen to me that was not foreseen by you and directed to my greater good from all eternity. This is enough for me.

I adore your holy, eternal and unfathomable designs. I submit to them with all my heart for love of you. I make a sacrifice of my whole being to you and join my sacrifice to that of Jesus, my divine Saviour.

In his name and by his infinite merits, I ask you to give me patience in my sufferings and perfect submission, so that everything you want or permit to happen will result in your greater glory and my sanctification. Amen.

FOR A SICK CHILD

The Daughter of the Canaanite Woman Healed

Jesus left that place and withdrew to the region of Tyre and Sidon. Then out came a Canaanite woman from that district and started shouting, 'Sir, Son of David, take pity on me. My daughter is tormented by a devil'. But he answered her not a word. And his disciples went and pleaded with him. 'Give her what she wants', they said, 'because she is shouting after us.' He said in reply: 'I was sent to the House of Israel.' But the woman had come up and was kneeling at his feet. 'Lord', she said, 'help me'. He replied: 'It is not fair to take the children's food and throw it to the house dogs.' She retorted: 'Ah yes, sir; but even house dogs can eat the scraps that fall from the master's table'. Then Jesus answered her: 'Woman, you have great faith. Let your wish be granted.' And from that moment her daughter was well again. (Mt. 15, 21-28)

Reflection Serious illness is always a difficult time for any of us. However, one of the things that is even more difficult is the serious illness of someone we love dearly. This is particularly true for parents when they see one of their children struck down. It is a time of great anxiety and confusion. It is also a time of anger at God and at life. It is above all else a time of feeling totally helpless, a time when they would willingly take onto themselves the sickness and pain of their loved one, but they know that this is not possible.

They are willing to go to any extreme to get a cure for this person who means so much to them.

That is the scene we are presented with in the story above. It can look harsh on the part of Christ who seemed to push this woman away from him. The point of the story, however, is the wonderful love she has for her daughter and the perseverance she shows in her search for healing. The faith that Jesus praises is not just her faith in him and what he can do for her. It is also very much the faith she shows in the depth of love she has for her daughter in which she only wants everything that is good and best for this little one. In this she becomes a model for what God is like in his love for each one of us.

Prayer   Creator God, you are both mother and father to us in your love and concern. Help us to believe more firmly in your love.

We ask your blessing on all those who are sick or suffering in any way. We pray especially for those who are suffering because of the illness of a loved one. Be with them and give them hope for the future.

We pray for all children who suffer serious illnesses. Give them strength to face the future and wisdom to understand the present. Be with their parents who also suffer greatly through this difficult time. And we remember those who take such good care of these children in our hospitals. Reward them for their goodness.

We pray for all our own loved ones who are sick at this time. Hear the love that is in our hearts for them and help us to know that this love is only a symbol of the love you have for them. Hear our prayers for them and bring them to healing and health.

May Mary, the Mother of Jesus your Son, and our Mother also, pray with us and for us in these difficult times of illness. We ask this through Christ, our Lord. Amen.

Psalm 8
How great is your name, O Lord our God,
through all the earth.

Your majesty is praised above the heavens.
On the lips of children and of babes
you have found praise to foil your enemy,
to silence the foe and the rebel.

When I see the heavens, the work of your hands,
the moon and the stars which you arranged,
What are we that you should keep us in mind
mortal flesh that you care for us.

Yet you have made us little less than gods;
with glory and honour you crowned us,
gave us power over the works of your hands
put all things under our feet.

How great is your name, O Lord our God,
through all the earth.

THE MEMORARE

Remember, O most gracious Virgin Mary, that never was it known that anyone who fled to your protection, implored your help or sought your intercession, was left unaided. Inspired with this confidence, I fly to you, O Virgin of virgins, my Mother. To you I come, before you I stand, sinful and sorrowful. O Mother of the Word Incarnate, despise not my petitions, but in your mercy hear and answer me. Amen.

WE ARE PRECIOUS IN HIS EYES
The Son of the Widow of Nain
Restored to Life

*Now soon afterwards Jesus went to a town called Nain,
accompanied by his disciples and a great number of people.
When he was near the gate of the town it happened that a dead
man was being carried out for burial, the only son of his mother,
and she was a widow. And a considerable number of townspeople
were with her. When the Lord saw her he felt sorry for her. 'Do
not cry,' he said. Then he went up and put his hand on the bier
and the bearers stood still, and he said, 'Young man, I tell you to
get up'. And the dead man sat up and began to talk, and Jesus
gave him to his mother. Everyone was filled with awe and praised
God saying, 'A great prophet has appeared among us; God has
visited his people'. And this opinion of him spread throughout
Judaea and all over the countryside. (Lk. 7, 11-19)*

Reflection Raising someone from the dead is a most extraordinary
event and all we can do is marvel at it. But it is the
promise of Jesus to all of us that we too will be raised to
life on the last day. However this story is not just about
Jesus bringing this young man back to life. It is rather
about Jesus restoring his mother to her proper dignity.
In the culture of the time, a woman who had no man
was regarded as almost a non-person. She had no
dignity in the community and, as well as coping with
the heartbreak of losing her son, she was going to have
to live without any prospects for the future.

Serious illness can also rob us of our dignity as we see life changed so dramatically and sometimes so suddenly. We can feel that we are useless, a burden to others, unable to do so many of the ordinary things of life, and we can despair. This story of healing is a reassurance to us that Christ, above all else, wants to assure us that we are precious in his eyes and to know also how precious we are in the hearts of all those who love us.

As you read this story, let Christ speak to your heart. Hear him speak his word, 'Do not cry.' Feel his touch, as he heals the parts of you that may have died because of your illness, those parts that may be your hope, your peace, your joy, your gratitude for all you have, your sense of your special dignity as a daughter or son of God.

Prayer God of love, you have created me in your own image and likeness and given me the dignity of being your daughter, your son. Be with me in this time of illness so that I can always know how precious I am in your eyes. Let me feel the presence of Christ your Son as he touches the parts of me that have died because of this illness, so that he can restore me to life. Help me to be renewed in hope and confidence. And through the touch of Christ may I know the peace that only he can bring, the peace that the world cannot give. Help me never to despair, but to trust always in your love. Amen.

Psalm 141

With all my voice I cry to the Lord,
with all my voice I entreat the Lord.
I pour out my trouble before him;
I tell him all my distress
while my spirit faints within me.
But you, O Lord, know my path.

I cry to you, O Lord.
I have said: 'You are my refuge,
all I have in the land of the living.'
Listen then to my cry
for I am in the depths of distress.

Rescue me from those who pursue me
for they are stronger than I.
Bring my soul out of this prison
and then I will praise your name.
Around me the just will assemble
because of your goodness to me.

COUNTING YOUR BLESSINGS
The Ten Lepers

On the way to Jerusalem Jesus travelled along the border between Samaria and Galilee. As he entered one of the villages, ten lepers came to meet him. They stood some way off and called to him, 'Jesus! Master! Take pity on us'. When he saw them he said, 'Go and show yourselves to the priests'. Now as they were going away they were cleansed. Finding himself cured, one of them turned back praising God at the top of his voice and threw himself at the feet of Jesus and thanked him. The man was a Samaritan. This made Jesus say. 'Were not all ten made clean? The other nine, where are they? It seems that no one has come back to give praise to God, except this foreigner.' And he said to the man, 'Stand up and go on your way. Your faith has saved you.' (Lk. 17, 11-19)

Reflection This well-known story helps us to understand the difference between a cure and a healing. All ten people were cured from their leprosy. Only one was healed, the one who came back to give praise to God and to Jesus who had made such a difference in his life. The other nine – and there is nothing in the story to indicate that they were all men! – went back to their ordinary lives and the only difference was that they no longer had leprosy. This one person had joy bubbling out of him. His whole life had been transformed.

Gratitude is one of the sure signs of being healed. And gratitude is possible even when we are suffering serious illness. This doesn't mean that we have to be grateful for being ill in some kind of fatalistic way. Rather it means that we can look beyond the illness and see all the wonderful gifts of life that are in us and around us and give thanks to God and to one another for all of these.

Sometimes a cure of our illness is possible and we should always pray for that for ourselves and for one another. Healing is always possible if we open ourselves up to the presence of Christ with us and to the love of God that is in us.

Prayer God of infinite love, I thank you for your love for me. Help me to believe ever more fully in your love so that my life may be filled with gratitude and tranquillity.

I thank you for the wonder of my being and the wonder of being alive. Help me, each day, to rejoice in the gift of life and to count my blessings.

I thank you for my mind through which I come to know you and to recognise the goodness of everything around me. Keep my mind alive to thoughts of goodness and greatness.

I thank you for my heart through which I can love you and the many loved ones in my life. Keep my heart alive to the joys of love and to the goodness of all those who love me.

I thank you for my soul through which I am destined for eternal life. Keep my soul young and fresh so that I can always celebrate life and have no fear of death.

I thank you for my body through which I enjoy the pleasures of life and feel the pains of life. Through the fragility of my body keep me aware that everything is a gift from you, the one who loves me with an infinite love, so that I may never lose your gift of peace even in the midst of suffering.

I thank you for the gift of faith through which all of this makes sense. Strengthen this gift in my life so that I can know that my sufferings may be added to the sufferings of Christ for the salvation of the world to the glory of your name. Amen.